I0439505

1

CURVY IS THE NEW THIN!
Published by
Chenai & Co. California © 2013

Printed in the United States of America

Curvy is the new thin!

A guide to a healthy, wholesome you!

In loving memory of my father,
Clemence Vama Muchemwa

Book editor~ Danai Salerno

Acknowledgment

Dear God, thank you for this opportunity to help those who are struggling with their weight. I pray you may release your children from negative thought patterns and self destructive eating habits that have put them in this predicament. I pray that as they follow this weight loss guide, the swan inside of them may emerge. Above all, I pray the struggle with weight ends, and makes way for the beauty in their hearts to shine forth.

Foreword

Hello and welcome curvy women! Are you tired of trying to fit in a box you just don't belong? If your mother and aunts are curvaceous, chances are you were never meant to be built like a boy! It is time to stop feeling ashamed about your hips, and butt, and boobs and instead embrace them. A woman's crown of glory are her hair and her curves! Growing up in Africa I witnessed many women who were very skinny, but still had their curves. Africa is usually portrayed as a poor continent, ravaged with illness and starvation.

However, Africa is a huge continent with so many cultures, tribes and languages. It is not only the cradle of civilization, but it holds centuries of traditions, and ancient practices that are valuable today. Africa holds some weight loss secrets that you can apply to your life today. The African standards of beauty embrace real women who have curves!

We are not here to obsess about calories, exclude certain food groups and exercise excessively.

With our help you can lose weight, and maintain when you reach your health goal. Above all, you will enjoy the journey of discovery, as much as we enjoyed sharing what we know with you. Thank you for joining us in this revolutionary thinking. Success to your weight loss! Don't lose the curves, rock your curves!

Curvy vs. Thin…

As a child growing up in Harare, my parents would send me to the garden in our backyard to pick fresh fruits and vegetables. Organic food was my constant companion. At the age of five, my parents planted a plum tree and put me in charge of it. Sadly, birds used to get to the plums way before I did. Now, even though I had more access to organic food than processed food, that is not the choice I made. For a long time, I happily munched on potato chips everyday. I even had ice cream and meat pies all the time. My weight gain happened progressively, gaining a few pounds each year, until I was fat at only ten years old. At the age of 13, I went to boarding school, grouped with other overweight teenagers and walked everyday before school. I lost so much weight; I became the talk of the school for a while. However, my father simply was unimpressed; he told me he worked too hard to have me looking thin, gaunt and hungry. "At least look healthy!" he begged me. My uncles told me to eat up because African men weren't interested in sticks with no meat. "Eat, child!" They liked to encourage, "You need your curves, trust us." They would say and then laugh. One uncle even bluntly told me that I was trying to attain the level of beauty of the western world, filled with starving and superficial women.

I didn't really listen to the advice, after all how many teenagers do you know who do?

Years later when I first arrived in Denton Texas, I noticed how easy it was to gain weight. You could gain weight, at an alarming rate. At the age of 20, I stood on the scale and jumped right off. What can I say; this was my form of denial. I couldn't believe it, I was 5"4 and just over 200 pounds!

 In Africa, the junk food wasn't loaded with Trans fats and corn syrup. In America portion sizes were so much bigger, and the food loaded with chemicals I couldn't pronounce, clearly I couldn't get away with happily munching on chips, and ice cream and pies. I tried many diets, most didn't last 3 days.

Finally, I sat down and wrote a plan that I knew would work for me. I lost 60 pounds, miraculously grew two inches taller, and have never gained the weight back. I am not one to exclude carbohydrates, obsess about calories and exercise excessively.

We all can learn from the ancient Agrarian lifestyle that was practiced by the average African citizen. This lifestyle is very simple, relaxed and above all fulfilling.

Curvy vs. Unhealthy

There is a thin line between being curvy and unhealthy!
You have to be in a healthy range! If your doctor warns you to lose weight, please do not deceive yourself. Please listen. You want to be toned and voluptuous. In Mauritania you find husbands who get upset when their women go on a diet and try to lose weight! We find women who are encouraged to be obese.
Here they believe obesity is a sign of wealth. This is an extreme way of thinking too. Bottom line is you have to be in your healthy range.

My grandparents lived long healthy lives. My grandfather died at the age of 105. He cooked for himself until only two weeks before his death. Grandfather, wore a suit everyday and went about his business. He ate healthy and was very active. My grandmother was a very petite, curvy woman. She too ate healthy, and loved outdoor activities. She died at 93. Both my grandparents ate carbohydrates everyday, and enjoyed wine and beer, occasionally. I learned from them to strive to live a happy, fulfilling life, not based on just looks. Curvy woman, it is time to step into the light and shine! Stop beating yourself up for not looking like a stick. You were not created to be that way anyway.

What is true Beauty?

Emotional states such as boredom, loneliness, anxiety and stress often drive people to eat mindlessly.
 Furthermore, being busy all the time and always living in a fast paced environment drives people to eat just to get through the day. We also live in a society that bombards us with flawless images of beauty and perfection contributing to low self esteem, and a trip to the refrigerator to ease feelings of worthlessness.

Consider this African folklore

Once upon a time in ancient Africa, deep in the jungle of the Mambo, lived an animal kingdom. The King was, of course, the Great Lion. Flanked on his right at most times was his elegant wife, Queen Lioness. All the animals went to the King Lion with their problems and he usually solved them.

However, one day baby Elephant approached the throne with a question." King Lion," he asked slowly, "why are my legs so wide, my skin so coarse, and why is my complexion a dull gray? I have noticed my sprint is not as effortless as yours and I wish I had a royal mane to shake like you do. Then you have such a lovely golden brown complexion that even the sun admires, for I have seen her rays dancing on you. Oh what I would do just to be you for a day! As for your nose, it is perfect. I have a trunk for a nose. I couldn't hide it if I tried."

The King Lion gasped at the obvious torture baby elephant was going through. He turned to his wife for support but she too appeared unsure. Luckily, Monkey came to the rescue.

"I have a potion your majesty that might settle this matter once and for all. Baby Elephant here needs to be a lion for as long as it takes before he comes to peace with who he is."

"Oh could you! Would you really transform me into a lion?"

"If His majesty approves, let me go ahead with this potion, I surely can. My magic is tried and true, and dates back to the land before time. I warn you baby elephant, if you really want this it can be done."
"Yes! Yes! I want to be a Lion!" Baby elephant raised his trunk and blew it in victory.

The Great King Lion roared loudly. When all was quiet, he proclaimed, "Let him have his way. Tomorrow you will be a lion!"
So it was that the next day, when baby elephant arose, he was a lion. Excitedly, he ran to the beautiful pools to stare at his reflection.
"Handsome!" he concluded. He was absolutely handsome. Elated, he walked around the jungle kingdom proudly.

However, as he walked, he noticed how long and graceful giraffe was. He admired how giraffe could just stretch her neck and eat leaves from the trees. Baby elephant wanted a longer neck. His neck just wasn't long enough. As he was caught on this line of thought, peacock greeted, "Well baby Elephant how do you feel in your new body?"
"Great!" Baby elephant exclaimed dancing around her gallantly.
"Oh isn't that nice, maybe you will stay a Lion forever then?"
"Mmm…Maybe," Baby Elephant agreed a distant look in his eye. His mind was working again; what if his neck was longer and his mane had the colors of the peacock?
All day he thought about it. He wanted to be the best he could, and Monkey should make it so.

At the end of the day he was back at King Lion's throne.

"How did your first day as a Lion go?" King asked expectantly.

"Good. Good but…"

King Lion regarded him through compassionate eyes.

"I wish my neck was longer like giraffe, and my mane as colorful as the beautiful peacock's feather." Lion was crestfallen. "What do want next, wings?" He boomed angrily.

"You don't understand! You don't know how hard it is for me!" Elephant wailed.

Lion roared; anguish weighing heavily on his heart.

"Let him have his way" Monkey advised in a whisper.

"Yes" the Queen spoke. "Give him what he wants."

"He chooses a difficult path. It doesn't have to be this way!" Lion pleaded.

"This is a path baby elephant has to travel to find his way" Monkey soothed.

Lion felt doubtful, "W\hat is this madness baby elephant is caught in? He is the largest land animal! Just look at the strength in his trunk and tusks. Look at his thick skin that allows him to get away with so many mud baths! I can't even take a mud bath, it would ruin my fur!" Lion shook his head sadly.

"Monkey" he ordered. "Trouble me no more with baby elephant's request. Give him whatever he wants."

Baby elephant couldn't believe his luck when monkey told him he could have whatever he

desired. Over the following months baby elephant got whatever look he wanted. Baby elephant was convinced he would be happy if he could just get the perfect look! Monkey soon ran out of the magic transforming potion. "It takes years to create this potion, and you have used it all" Monkey explained. "Oh no what shall I do?" Baby elephant wailed. "What about, my dear? Over the past months you have added everything you could think of" Baby elephant paced restlessly. "Then why do I feel empty? Why do I feel so alone? I just wanted a piece of every animal added to myself, to make me more beautiful. I miss taking mud baths with the other elephants, then drying myself with my trunk. I miss eating grass, meat drives me crazy." Baby elephant walked to a pool nearby and stared at his reflection. "The other animals laugh at me openly especially hyena and crow. Constantly I am reminded of all I left behind. I would do anything to be an elephant again!" A tear dropped from baby elephant's face. "You said I could be an elephant again monkey. Turn me into an elephant again!"
"You know I certainly have run out of magic potions for you. However, there is a way you can be an elephant again."
Baby elephant pleaded. "What is it, tell me! I need to know!"
"You need to love the body you are in."
"That doesn't make any sense."
"You made some mistakes in your pursuit of outer beauty baby elephant. When you have truly forgiven yourself, and learned to love who you are, then a miracle will happen."

Elephant listened thoughtfully. He fell silent considering monkey's suggestion. Finally he announced. "I will start by going to King Lion. I think I owe him an apology. Then I need to apologize to my family and friends for the pain I caused them as I pranced around proudly like a lion and wanted nothing to do with them." Baby elephant sighed heavily. "I was so desperate to be beautiful. I really thought my life would change. I figured if I fixed myself on the outside, I would automatically change inside. Now I see it was the other way around. If I had truly loved myself, I would have been the happiest elephant in the kingdom." Monkey smiled happily. "Indeed I assure you, a miracle is on the way."

Baby elephant is no different from people who have undergone plastic surgery countless times in pursuit of beauty. Baby elephant's story reflects our struggles, as we go through life wishing we were just like the other person, yet this cannot be so. Each of us is unique!

The Curvy woman's guide to her best body...

The role of herbs and spices

Africa is home to many herbs and spices, because of the sub tropical and tropical climates prevalent throughout the continent. Years ago, hunters would collect different herbs and take them home to experiment with. Spices and herbs aided with the digestion of food. As African civilization progressed, herbs and spices were actually sown in the local village gardens. Spices and herbs regularly used had the beneficial effects of boosting the immune system and were a source of antioxidants. Recently, the herb Hoodia Gordonii has become popular in America. Hoodia Gordonii is a leafless spiny succulent plant found in South Africa and Namibia. For years Hoodia was used by Bushmen to suppress appetite when making long hunting trips. Just to name one of the most widely known.

Earth offers the good carbohydrates

Root vegetables are the main source of carbohydrates, such turnips, beets, carrots and sweet potatoes. Africans use the native potatoes which are smaller than the commercial potatoes, but contains twice the amount of protein. In some parts whole wheat grains are the main source of carbohydrates. Whole grains are richer in fiber, antioxidants and protein, vitamins (niacin, vitamin B6 and vitamin E) and dietary minerals (phosphorus, manganese and selenium). In Algeria the national dish is couscous (pasta made of crushed and steamed semolina).

Food preparation remains old fashioned

Most African food is steamed, boiled, roasted grilled or smoked. Fast food chains are few and therefore not popular. Instead you see local restaurants selling freshly prepared healthy foods. People enjoy sharing food at home or at friend's house. Africans are aware of the unhealthy ingredients in most prepackaged foods.

Access to better selection of meat and fish

Meat and meat products are consumed in moderation. Due to economic restraints, meat is not a staple in many areas. Meat is mostly used as an additive to soups, stews and salads. In Africa the livestock is grass-fed and this nourishes the body more. This is much better than growth stimulated and antibiotic force feed meats. When animals are properly raised they are an excellent source of protein and other nutrients like vitamins A, B and D. Fish and seafood, are consumed more than meat. They are the gift from nearby oceans, and rivers. In Ethiopia, Tilapia is popular because it is available. In South Africa, hake is popular because it is available. Healthy diets include fish oil because it is an excellent source of Omega 3 fatty acids. Fish oil regulates cholesterol in the body

A great appreciation for fruits, legumes and vegetables

High consumption of fruits, legumes (beans, peas) and vegetables is commonplace. Meals consist of a delightful mixture of vegetables, fruits and legumes. In Rwanda and Burundi beans are eaten for breakfast, lunch and dinner.

Lovely berries

Africans eat plenty of berries like raspberries, blueberries, blackberries, strawberries, cranberries, marion berries and boysenberries. Berries are rich in antioxidants and low in calories. In America, berry based nutrition drinks are very popular; for instance, the Goji and Acai berry drinks.

Natural sweeteners

Sugar was not a part of the Ancient African diets until late in history. Honey was used as sweetener. Honey was also used to clean burns and wounds. Africans still eat honeycomb and honey as a snack. It is easier for them to locate the bees' hives thanks to an amazing bird called the Honey Guide. The Honey Guide feeds on bees, bee-larvae and honeycomb. Most people used various fruits as sweeteners. You will be surprised how sweet natural grown fruit can taste when you limit refined white sugar. In ancient times, salt was obtained from various plants and the sea. (Unrefined sea salt) Still today Africans salt is a filtrate of ashes from banana peels, water reeds, sorghum head, dry leaves and normal ash.

Good oils

Consumption of saturated fat oils and Trans fats (hydrogenated oils) is low. Africans use minimally processed, beneficial oils like Argan oil, Peanut oil, and Olive oil.

The hunter gatherer lifestyle

Historically, Africans are hunter gatherers. Therefore, exercise is incorporated daily. There is no need for rigorous exercise plans. Nuts and dried fruits are collected by women and children, while men hunt for wild meat. To this day nuts are used to flavor various dishes. Africa holds many secrets to using common foods in un-American uncommon ways to create a healthy balanced diet.

Meals are lively social events

Most Africans use their hands to eat their food. Meals are long, enjoyable social events. This slows down eating and gives them time to chew food thoroughly before swallowing. It takes at least 5 minutes for your stomach to send a signal to your brain telling it, it is full.

Siesta!

Unlike most cultures, lunch is the main meal of the day. Eating a light breakfast of high energy nutritious, fibrous foods allows for productive mornings. Africans usually take afternoon naps widely known as siestas. They rest for about two hours after enjoying lunch.

Joyful dancing and singing

Dancing and singing are at the heart and soul of the African lifestyle. The beating of the drum in any village community evokes so many emotions. The drum is the sign of life in Africa, giving a sense of belonging and solidarity. Dancing is used to teach social patterns and values. Singing helps people work. Both dancing and singing are used to celebrate weddings, funerals, reciting, poetry, proverbs or history. Dancing is even used spiritually to encounter the "other world." The health benefits of dancing are mental and physical. Dancing generally provides a good cardiovascular workout. If the dancing focuses on core muscles it may increase flexibility and strength.

The benefits of plant based products

Africans use plant based skin products. For instance, the egg shaped nut of Shea trees. The Shea nut produces a solid vegetable fat used to enhance the taste, and texture of food. When added to your diet, Shea butter produces changes in digestion and aids greatly in weight loss. Shea butter is used as an ingredient for skin products globally. Another popular plant based skin product is cocoa butter. Cocoa butter is an edible fat extracted from the cacao bean. Cocoa butter is used to make chocolate. In ancient Africa, chocolate was mostly a beverage and had nothing to do with sugar. Minerals, antioxidants, and natural fat were found in various chocolate and cocoa products. The benefits of chocolate were embraced and even warriors used it for strength and to fight fatigue. Chocolate was considered a food vital for health. Sadly, over the centuries, chocolate has lost its medicinal and nutritional as more milk and sugar has been added to it. Dangerous toxins can be introduced in the body through the products we use for our skin. For overall health Africans eat Bitter leaf. Bitter leaf is a variety of African greens. It is used medicinally, to fight intestinal parasites.

Bitter leaf is soaked and washed before cooking to reduce the bitter taste.

Traditional homemade drinks

My grandparents used to make a tamarind drink. They also made their own home-made beer which was very common in their village. Traditional beers are made from various kinds of millet, sorghum, corn, or plantains. Sodas, and other processed sweet beverages are not consumed daily, but saved for specific occasions.

Water, tea and coffee, are the drinks of choice to most Africans. Africans use hot tea and coffee, to cut through the fat of a potentially greasy meal. In Morocco tea is the national drink. In Ethiopia, coffee is the national drink. Ethiopians can be found enjoying coffee for hours after their meals. (The coffee is not loaded with sugar and cream!) Drinking warm or hot tea with meals avoids fat in foods solidifying. Cold water solidifies the oil in our food and therefore slows digestion. In ancient times tribesmen would take the coffee berries on hunting trips mixed with other food staples. The berry was used to satiate the appetite. For centuries Africans have made their own wine and beer. Palm wine is a favorite in West Africa. In Ethiopia you find a wine made from honey, called Tej. In Central Africa, among the Mbuti people, a beverage called liko is found, made from berries, herbs and kola nuts.

Minimally processed dairy products

The traditional African diet has a moderate intake of milk and dairy products. Milk is obtained from organic fed cows, goats and sheep to make cheese, butter and yogurt. Milk and milk products are minimally processed.

Unique secondary source of protein

Green leafy vegetables are considered a secondary source of protein. Boiled greens like amaranth are an excellent source of protein, vitamin C, iron and calcium. Spinach, kale, Swiss chard, and collard greens are widely grown and consumed. Green leafy vegetables are usually added to stews, soups, casseroles, and side dishes. Almost every main meal is served with green leafy vegetables.

Ultimately, Africans eat plenty of food that was enjoyed in ancient times. Gifts of the sea and gifts from the earth! For instance, African red rice, and cowpeas were cultivated in the Mediterranean region in ancient times. They have been grown for centuries all over Africa. The basic cooking methods used to prepare the African cuisine can be traced back to ancient times.

Eating Like the Ancients

This section will help you to identify Western eating habits that may be working against your weight loss plan. Recent food inventions in Western nations, served to introduce more highly processed foods. The staple food in Western nations such as fast foods, (fried foods) convenience foods, canned foods, salty snacks, and meats have gained popularity. Considering the declining health of Western nations, African eating habits are far more beneficial for the body. African traditional diets are virtually free of heart disease, cancer, and other degenerative diseases and have sustained generations of healthy eating patterns.

This short questionnaire will assist you in identifying healthy diet changes:

What is in your refrigerator?

    a. I have all of the things that I love to eat?

    b. I only buy healthy fruits and snacks?

    c. I eat out most of the time the refrigerator is for drinks?

If you answered:

    a. You are closer to the right track than you think. In Africa most villagers go to the local farmers market every day to purchase fresh produce. However, they stock up on non-perishable foods weekly or bi-weekly. Having the things that you love to eat available in the home is economically sound.

The trick is to change what you love to eat. Stock up on natural whole foods and minimally processed foods.

b. Hopefully, you are on the right track. Be careful when you purchase "Healthy" snacks. Make sure they are not loaded with hidden calories and sugar. Select a variety of food that is high in fiber, delicious and nutritious.

c. Although eating out is a luxury in most parts of Africa, in Western nations dining at restaurants is a lifestyle. Some restaurant food can be unhealthy. The food is loaded with sodium, hidden calories, and saturated fats. Even vegetables might be loaded with butter and sodium! Nothing beats fresh homemade food! At least you know the food additives going into your dish. Choose the restaurants that at least offer a "healthy" menu. However, dining out too often will certainly slow you weight loss. Try to set a limit and have just one meal from a restaurant.

What is in your refrigerator and cabinets that you could pull from a garden?

a. I have mostly pre-packed and processed foods.

b. I have plenty of canned fruits and vegetables

c. I prefer fresh fruits and frozen vegetables

If you answered:

a. Pre-packed foods contain unhealthy levels of hydrogenated oils and additives. Certain food additives are considered potential carcinogens (a cancer causing substance or agent.) and are best avoided. Processed and smoked meat contains nitrates, which are known carcinogens. Prepackaged food also has high levels of sodium. MSG (Monosodium Glutamate) is an additive which is considered a flavor enhancer. Even some various food colorings are potential carcinogens. Bottom line preservatives aren't good for you. They can drive up your blood pressure and attribute to many other health problems. It's much better to get fresh foods.

b. Canned fruits and vegetables are a good option if you don't have fresh produce. Although canned fruits and vegetables have fewer nutrients, they can be combined creatively with other healthy dishes.

c. Find out where your local farmers' market is! This is a great way to shop for fresh produce, and spend time with your family. Fresh tender vegetables straight from the garden (or farmers' market) are best for freezing. You can wash, pack, seal and freeze your own vegetables. Purchasing frozen vegetables is a good option too. This means you can enjoy vegetables that are out of season.

What is your biggest meal of the day?

a. Breakfast

b. Lunch

c. Dinner

If you answered:

a. There has always been a link between breakfast and weight loss. A nutritious, balanced breakfast rich in protein and carbohydrates is a good way to start the day. Eating breakfast promotes blood level stability, more energy and helps with concentration. Your body needs breakfast to keep your energy levels high throughout the day!

b. Lunch should certainly be bigger than dinner! After all, you are more active during the day and are likely to burn off more calories.

c. Eating a big meal too late at night is a bad idea because you are less active and you don't burn the calories. Usually people who eat late at night, skip breakfast and lunch! This is very bad for the metabolism.

Do you feel you have enough time to sit and enjoy lunch? Do you bring lunch from home?

a. Yes, I plan my lunch and have at least 30 minutes to enjoy my lunch.

b. No, I just grab something from a nearby restaurant and try and eat it as fast as possible.

c. It depends on how I feel. Sometimes, I plan my lunch. Sometimes I just go out and buy something. I certainly don't take my full 30 minute lunch because of my workload.

If you answered:

    a. Taking time to actually enjoy your lunch, and chewing the food slowly savoring the taste is very important. Planning delicious meals ahead is essential, focusing on fat burning foods like lean protein, whole grains, light dairy and grapefruits. Drinking green tea with your warm lunch raises your metabolism.

b. Eating out is convenient but not necessarily healthy. Recent studies show that even the low fat restaurant menus, are high in calories, carbohydrates, and have artificial preservatives and additives.
Restaurant food is also a source of trans fat.
Trans fat is an additive you don't want to be feasting on. Trans fats may shorten your life (lower your good cholesterol and build bad cholesterol) even though they add the shelf life of food.
Wolfing down your food is bad. It leaves you unsatisfied and hungry.

    c. You could use this to your advantage. Adding variety to your eating plan is good. Taking care of your body should be your first priority. You deserve to sit down and forget working for at least 30 minutes. A stressful lifestyle could hinder weight loss.

How do you feel after lunch? Are you snacking on anything even after lunch?

a. I feel drowsy and tired after lunch.

b. I feel unsatisfied after lunch and can't wait until dinner. I snack mindlessly until I finally get home.

c. I have a hearty lunch and do not think about dinner.

If you answered:

    a. Your lunch is rich in simple carbohydrates that are low in fiber and raise your blood levels. High carbohydrate food can raise blood glucose levels. This triggers the synthesis and release of insulin. Too much insulin can cause health problems, such as obesity, and high blood pressure.

b. Lean protein will not raise your blood levels. Protein takes a while to digest and slows down digestion of the whole meal.

Lean protein also leaves you feeling fuller longer. This prevents you from snacking mindlessly on junk food, the rest of the day. Emotional instability is likely to lead us to mindless snacking. Loneliness, depression, and stress are some of the things that might be driving you to eat. Another cause of food cravings is adrenal fatigue. Stressors like insomnia, relationship issues, poor nutrition, and dieting, results in the adrenals dysfunction. This leads to adrenal fatigue and the body sends signals which we see as symptoms.

Some of the symptoms are: craving for carbohydrates, sugar or salt, reliance on stimulants, and weight gain.

c. If you are having a lunch that leaves you satisfied until your next snack time, good job!

Curvy woman, how far did you travel for food?

Agrarian Lifestyle Definition:

(Relating to land or land tenure. Pertaining to farmers or agricultural groups. Rural or agricultural.)

Most of the time we have no idea what journey the food we eat has been on. In Africa the journey food makes from the tree, or garden, or barn to the cooking pot, is not long. In fact 80% of the time you can actually trace the source of your food.

This is because the agricultural sector is the most important in Africa.

Africans pursue an Agrarian lifestyle that is simpler, home based, and organic. Life is less stressful.

Forget treadmills and hours of strenuous exercise after putting in eight hours of work. If you follow an Agrarian lifestyle, you are constantly moving, and therefore getting your daily exercise. The reason diets fail is because we have an unrealistic expectation of what our bodies should look like. The goal is to be healthy, well rested and happy. The goal is not to look flawless and perfect like most people we see on magazine covers. Having said that, weight loss secrets do not lie in counting and obsessing about calories. Nor do they lie in jumping on scales every morning, and scheming up daily or monthly often harmful, even fruitless crash diets.

Intuitively, we know it isn't healthy to be up at midnight, feasting on brownies and ice cream. Then when the brownies and ice cream show up in our bodies as excess weight we call for a quick remedy, and yet there isn't one. Losing weight in a short space of time only to gain it again is quite depressing.

If you adopt an Agrarian mindset, you are on the path to health.

To illustrate, imagine you are in an African village, what would you have for breakfast? Perhaps you would have fruits, nuts, goat cheese and perhaps a glass of milk. This is a far cry from doughnuts, and other calorie loaded fast food breakfast items. Fruits, nuts and cheese will go a long way to nourish the body.

In the village you won't find prepackaged foods, or restaurant chains and franchises. You don't find refrigerators either. Only the local butcher has a refrigerator…sometimes. As a result, food is always fresh. The meat that can't be used right away is cured, smoked, and stored as beef jerky. In Africa you will find a great selection of natural foods that your body really craves and needs. Think of yourself, as a hunter gatherer. What you are hunting for is the body God created in its perfection. The body you had before you subjected it to all the wrong food. You want to gather only the information that can help you.

Definition of Organic Food:

(Food grown without the use of fertilizers, sewage sludge, and human waste).

Organic food is not processed, and does not contain food additives. The livestock is grass fed. It is not reared with routine use of growth hormones and antibiotics.

Ancient Answer to Modern Problems

How much of the food you consume in a day is organic?

> A. I have no idea if the food I have is organic or not.

B. I find organic food is more expensive. I purchase organic food when I can.

C. I live nearby an organic store and the prices are good. Most of the food I enjoy is organic.

If you answered:

a. Find your local farmers' market, and shop there for fruits and vegetables. Replace prepackaged foods with fresh produce. Check the label when you purchase meat to see if it grass fed.

b. Some organic stores are more expensive than others. Select the one that will work with your budget. Also check your mail for weekly flyers from organic stores, so you can be aware of any sales they have.

c. Fortunately, there are some people who live right by affordable organic stores. Always keep your eye out for the weekly specials!

Definition of Dieting:

(To regulate the food a person eats, so as to improve physical condition.)

Sometimes the process of limiting food intake works for a certain period of time.

1. What was the last diet you tried and why did it fail?

Curvy woman denial will not get you the results you need! If your weakness is French fries, or chocolate, just indulge once in a while. Afterwards, drink plenty of water, and schedule a brisk walk for an hour on same day. The goal is to have a long period of time pass by before you have a craving. Just try not to overeat when you do.

Why Lunch is the Main Meal?

Africans follow the Agrarian lifestyle and begin the day as early as 4:00am in the morning. I remember one planting season when I was in the village. Grandpa and Grandma were up at 3:30am to wake everyone up, eat breakfast and go to the fields. The idea was to work when it was cool so when it was unmercifully hot, no one had to work. I always stayed behind with the other females to prepare lunch because it was the main meal of the day. When all my hardworking family returned from the fields, they were exhausted and famished. We, on the other hand had lunch ready to serve. Everyone sat down and took the time to actually enjoy the food. After lunch we all retreated for a two hour nap (siesta). Late in the afternoon we worked on completing various domestic chores. In the evening we snacked on beef jerky, various dried nuts, and legumes.

We all have an idea of what lunch is. For some, lunch is a bag of chips and a soda. For others it is four slices of pizza and soda.

Planning meals is very important. Having lunch as your main meal doesn't rob you of a delicious dinner. Just make lighter choices in the evening. Give your stomach a break!

I have met people who skip breakfast, skip lunch, then start eating late in the afternoon, and carry on till past midnight. This is not acceptable. I have also met people who don't drink water at all. All meals are very important. If you choose to have a beverage with your meal, we suggest you give it some thought. Cold water solidifies the oil in our food and therefore slows digestion. If your meal is hot, have warm water or beverage after.

Save the Best for Last...mmm Desserts

Desserts are typically at the end of the meal because they are usually so high in sugar and fat. The whole point of dessert is to give you closure. I love dessert. Sometimes I wish it was the main meal. However, I know this will not help my weight loss plan. In African cities fruit cake is very popular and served at weddings. The cakes are full of dried fruits (like raisins) and nuts.

If you're serious about losing weight forget enjoying dessert and or "junk food" 24/7. Chances are if you are overweight you have had your fair share. Cut your dessert and junk food intake to once a week. You can choose all natural, chips, cookies, brownies, cakes and ice cream which are available at your local healthy store.

The Paradox of Exercise

We know we need to exercise to help reach our weight loss goals. Truthfully, most people struggle with exercising. I have joined gyms only to cancel my membership a few months later. I have bought equipment that I use for a week or two before giving up. What I have found most challenging is exercising after a full eight to ten hour work day. The only exercise I have done consistently and enjoyed is yoga. Pick an exercise you enjoy!

In Africa gym enrollment is very low and even non-existent in rural parts. Following an Agrarian lifestyle means adequate exercise for the average African citizen. In rural areas exercise is just part of the daily routine. You have to go to the well to draw water. You have to walk to the garden to pick fresh produce or walk to the nearest farmers market.

When you see buses in the village, they are usually on long distance routes. Food prep is time consuming and a good form of exercise. For instance, people make their own peanut butter, and corn meal. The barn animals have to be fed, and taken for walks so they too can get adequate air and exercise.

In the cities some people who live on the outskirts choose to walk to work, even when they own cars, just for the exercise. My uncle walks everyday to town and he owns two cars. My mother is a nurse and she goes gardening to get her daily exercise. She really treasures her flowers and plants in her backyard.
If you want to lose weight choose to walk at every opportunity you get. If you get two 15 minute breaks at work, why not take a walk, especially if you work in an office and are sitting at your desk all day. If you get an hour lunch, take some time to walk.
Walk briskly and frequently, and you will find your body rests well when you finally go to sleep. One of the best workouts is walking up and down a flight of stairs for 20 minutes about three times a week. You will love how this lifts your assets!

If you want to tone your body, while having fun, go join a dance class! If you have on exercise on demand, dance in your home! Africans get most of their exercise from dancing. Traditional African dance tell the stories of ancient cultures. Traditional dances are often performed during celebrations. Therefore, onlookers are encouraged to take part in the dance as well. Usually, men and women have very different steps to learn and the choreography is exact.

There are many forms of Traditional African dance which are listed below.

Love Dances: Dance may be used to narrate a love story. This dance is usually performed at weddings. In Ghana the women perform the Nmane dance at weddings in honor of the bride.

Healing Dances: The traditional healing dance draws inspiration from nature. Healing dances move you physically and emotionally, as you celebrate life and become one with nature.

Warriors Dances: The warrior dance is performed before and after battles. Shaka

Zulu the great African warrior and King, made his warriors dance on thorny ground to make them tough for battle. The Zulu warrior dance is regarded as the touchstone of Zulu identity. This warrior dance is well choreographed with perfect precision and timing. It is danced by men of any age dressed in animal skin, head rings, ceremonial belts, ankle rattles, shields and weapons. Dancers make mock stabs at imaginary enemies.

Rites of Age and Coming of Age Dances: These dances are performed to mark the coming of age. The Zulu Reed dance is an educational experience for young girls to learn how to behave before the King. The girls wear beads, which is a mark of African beauty. Sometimes they wear rattles made of seedpods around the ankles. The rite of passage and coming of age dances give confidence to the dancers as they perform in front of everyone.

Welcome Dances: Welcome dances are often highly spirited accompanied by rhythmic drums. They serve to welcome visitors, and at the same time display the hosts' talent and spirit of generosity.

Possession and Summoning Dances: This traditional dance where Africans try to summon spirits, in animals, plants or ancestors.

Spiritual Dances: This is when Africans dance to a prayer, and call forth blessings.

Africa home of curvy women!

Africa ~ Territories, History & Cuisine

The Southern African Cuisine

Territories:

Zimbabwe
Angola
Botswana
Lesotho
Malawi
Mozambique
Madagascar
Namibia
South África
Swaziland
Zambia

History and Food:

Southern Africans were mostly hunter-gatherers. The mild-climate and abundance of rain allowed for tropical fruit such as mangoes, bananas, and pineapple to grow.

Southern Africans would gather foods like squash, coconuts, fresh fruits and dried fruits. They raised their own cattle, chickens, goats and lamb. Dried, salted, and spiced meat called biltong (similar to jerky) became a very popular food.

As the years progressed the Southern African countries were colonized by western powers from Europe. The practice of modern agriculture was introduced, and Southern Africans were taught to grow vegetables, such as corn and sweet potatoes. Trade also increased as more Western powers settled.

Trade was between Africa, Europe and India. This brought diversity of spices, herbs and recipes that influenced the local diet. However, curry was loved the most.

You will find dishes of European or Asian origin prepared the Southern African way. For instance, the chicken, beef and lamb pot pies contain fruits, nuts and of course curry powder. Well seasoned beef sausages are very popular too and are served with main meals. The best sausages are wrapped in steak, (instead of casings) then roasted in the oven. The tamarind fruit is native to Africa, and is cultivated throughout the Southern African region. It is known for its cathartic properties (helps digestion) and was used in ancient times as a medicine. It was also used to lower body temperature. In Southern Africa it is found in various Indian based curries, chutneys and British Worcestershire sauce. The tamarind drink is made by combining the seeds with water and sugar cane.

Stews are enjoyed in most villages. Food is simmered in three legged iron pots over open fire for hours.
Different ingredients are added depending on what is available in the garden at the time.
In Landlocked countries such as Zimbabwe, Zambia, Swaziland, and Botswana you find subsistence farmers. (farmers that grow only enough food to feed their families. They may occasionally go to the markets to supplement their diets.) Due to economic restraints, meat is not consumed every meal. Goat, sheep and cattle found on subsistence farms are used for milk, cheese, butter, yogurt, fuel, and wool.
Corn and sorghum are used to create various dishes like sadza, (maize ground into a fine meal, which is cooked in water until it has the consistency of mashed potato.) mealie meal corn soup, mutakura (mixture of boiled corn and peanuts) and corn meal porridge.
Seafood is a staple food in the parts of Southern Africa, along the Atlantic and Ocean coastlines. Hake is the most common fish,

caught in the Atlantic Ocean waters. The ocean also offers a variety of other seafood like shrimp, calamari, tuna, lobster and mackerel.

Traditional beers are made from various kinds of maize, millet, sorghum, or plantains. Homemade beers are popular and may vary slightly in each village. Beer is brewed (that is heated before fermentation) and ginger or fruit may be added to it to suit the creator's taste.

The San are the bushmen found in the Kalahari desert. The San have lived there for about 20,000 years. Historically, they are nomadic hunter gatherers. The San survive by hunting for game, like antelope, kudu, and birds. The San diet consists mainly of highly nutritious edible plants like melons and berries. The famous Hoodia Gordonii, miracle appetite suppressant is found in the Kalahari desert. The women usually gather the fruits, nuts, vegetables and other edible plants. The Mongongo nuts are their staple food because they grow everywhere in this area and are high in protein (26 grams). The Mongongo nut oil is used as a skin rub that provides protection from the harsh hot environment. The nut also has other nutrients like calcium, iron, zinc, magnesium, and thiamine. It also has high concentration of vitamin E.

Traditional Dancing:

Traditional dance is used as a form of cultural expression. Traditional costumes made of animal skins are worn when dancing. In Zimbabwe we find the Muchongoyo dance used at weddings, or rituals. Shaking hoshas (a musical instrument, a gourd with seeds inside) and beating rhythmic drums are at the heart of the Muchongoyo dance. The men's dance involves high knee lifts. The women shake the hoshas and dance around the drummers and the men.

In Zambia girls and boys spend months practicing in seclusion the dance for the coming of age rituals. The African rumba is also very popular in Southern Africa. The details differ, but this exercise impacts the lower body the most.

The Northern African Cuisine

Territories:

Algeria
Egypt
Libya
Sudan (parts of)
Tunisia
Morocco
Western Sahara
Mauritania

History and Food:

North Africa lies along the Mediterranean sea. The North African countries include Egypt, Morocco, Tunisia and Algeria. There is so much culinary diversity, because for centuries travelers, traders, migrants and immigrants influenced the diet. The food shows influences of Arabs, Berber, Turks and French tastes. Potatoes, chilies, zucchini, and tomatoes came with outside influence. Olive oil has long been at the heart of North African dishes. Most of them have the same dishes prepared slightly differently and given a different name. The dishes are very flavorful, because they are prepared with a variety of spices like, cinnamon, coriander, cumin, dill, fennel, cloves, garlic, ginger, and saffron. The North African countries, especially Egypt, are thought to have had better food than many others in the ancient world. Ancient Egypt was blessed with rich, dark fertile soil, and its proximity to the Nile river. Agriculturally Ancient Egyptians diet consisted of breads, poultry, fruits, dairy products, and fish. They made breads in tall ovens with fireboxes at the bottom. Sometimes beans, dried fruits and vegetables were added to the breads. The vegetables consumed often, were lettuce, leeks, green beans, beans, chickpeas, and lentils. Tomatoes were a popular ingredient in most dishes. Fruits like dates and grapes (or dried grapes in the form of raisins) were used as sweeteners. Dates are rich in both sugar and protein.

Morocco is considered to have some of the healthiest dishes. Moroccan dishes are flavored with turmeric, saffron, cumin, oregano, thyme, coriander, chili powder, parsley, cinnamon; onion and garlic Moroccans consume more fish and seafood than the other Northern African countries. Fish has easily digestible protein, and contains essential fats, minerals and vitamins. Fish is a good source of polyunsaturated fatty acids, especially omega-3 fatty acids. Moroccans also rely on whole wheat grain products (breads, pasta) high in fiber and vitamins and nutrients.

Tea (green and mint tea) also is an important part of the Moroccan culture and is widely consumed with food. It is believed tea was first introduced in the 18th century by European and Asian traders. China was the main provider of green tea. The methods of preparing Moroccan tea vary and can be complex.

Morocco is home to the argania spinosa tree and the fruits are used to make argan oil. Chefs are known to use argan oil for preparing gourmet healthy meals. Argan oil has a unique composition. It is rich in antioxidants, and essential fatty acids, and high levels of vitamin E. Studies show it protects against cardiovascular disease, inflammatory disorders and even prevents skin cancer. Traditionally, women have used it for their skin, hair and nails.

Tunisians' meals are long social events and time is set aside to enjoy meals. Seafood and fish are available in great abundance and variety, thanks to the nearby sea. Freshly baked whole grain bread is available every day and is served at each meal. A typical meal may begin with soup, followed by fish or seafood salad. The main meal usually consists

of stews and lamb roasts, vegetables and
cheese.
Dessert consists of coffee, tea, salads, fruits,
custards and thin pastries.

The Sahara desert is the largest in the world.
The Sahara Desert covers eighty percent of
the land in Algeria. There you find desert
nomads who are constantly moving from
place to place, in search of water, food and
grazing lands. Desert nomads carry, dates,
nuts, and rice. From their animals they get
cheese, yogurt, butter, and meat.

Traditional Dancing:

Belly dancing or Egyptian dance is native to
North Africa. Some believe it originates from
the indigenous dances of ancient upper Egypt.
The Egyptian dance is a visual expression of
joy, as generations of women dance together
uniquely moving their bodies in time to the
music. Costumes worn are designed according
to the type of belly dance. Neighboring
Tunisia and Morocco adopted the belly dance
with variations like using scarves and baskets.
The Nubian dance culture has been passed
from generation to generation. It involves a lot
of drum beat and clapping. The Nubian
Egyptian belly dance remains popular even
today.

The Western African Cuisine

Territories:

Liberia
Mali
Niger
Nigeria
Senegal
Sierra Leone
Togo
Benin
Burkina Fasco
Cameroon
The Gambia
Ghana
Guinea
Guinea-Bissau

History and Food:

Fufu - Any dish made by boiling any sort of flour; maize (corn) cassava, sorghum, or millet.

Typical western meals are very flavorful, and full of chilies, peppers, and other hot spices. It is the kind of hot food that makes you sweat.

Hot spicy food can give a kick to your heart rate. There is historic influence from Arabs, who they traded with. Arabs introduced mint, cloves, and cinnamon. Yams are widely consumed in West Africa. Countries along the coast like Nigeria and Cameroon have varieties of yam.

The cuisines are prepared with fufu which is made from root vegetables, such as yams, coco yams, or cassava. Fufu is sometimes made from cereal grains or plantains. In certain parts of West Africa, like Liberia and Mauritania rice is a staple. Meat, fish, vegetables, legumes, and fruit are prepared in very creative ways. Beans are ground, mixed with onions, tomatoes, and eggs then made into cakes. Root vegetables are usually mashed and added to stews, and soups. Sweet plantains are boiled or ground to make fufu. Sometimes sweet plantains are fried. Seafood and meat are often combined. Seafood is plentiful and is combined with beef, chicken or goat or lamb. Some fish is left to dry then lightly fried with peppers, onions and tomatoes. Most cooks use pineapple, citrus fruits, black eyed peas, okra, sweet potatoes, rice, peanuts, yams, green peas, cereal grains and coco yams.

Peanuts are widely cultivated and enjoyed in West Africa. Traditional dishes utilize the peanut in various ways. Before the peanut was introduced to Africa by Europeans the Bambara groundnut was popular. The peanut replaced the Bambara groundnut, because of their similarity. Peanut oil is for cooking and flavoring food. The palm tree family found in West Africa is a gift. From the tree comes the nut that is used to make red palm oil, and palm butter. Africans use palm oil and butter to make stews, sauces, soups and many other dishes.

Coconut palm trees are valuable in many ways. Africans make the coconut wine from the sap by allowing it to ferment. They also make vinegar and gel from the sap. The fruit is used for water and juice. The leaves are used to make firewood, brooms, baskets, thatch roofs and even palm cabbage. Palm cabbage is eaten as a vegetable.
Coconut oil is used for cooking. Extra virgin coconut oil is used for weight loss. It is an antidote against obesity and diabetes.
Coconut milk is used to flavor food. Coconut milk is obtained from the meat of a mature coconut.

A different way Africans grill and steam their food is by using leaves. Food like fish, meat & vegetables are wrapped in banana leaves or other certain types of leaves. (depending on what flavor they give the food) The leaves are grilled over hot coals or steamed in a pot.

Traditional Dancing:

There are many types of dances found in West Africa. Moribayasa is a dance; the name originating from a tree that grows near a village in Guinea. The dance is designed to break the pattern of bad luck. The woman experiencing bad luck wears ragged, dirty clothes and dances around the tree to the beating of drums and prayerful song. Afterwards, she removes the dirty, ragged clothes and buries them.

The Eastern African Cuisine

Territories:
Tanzania
Somalia
Kenya
Burundi
Rwanda
Ethiopia
Eritrea
Djibouti
Uganda
Sudan (parts of)

History and Food:

In Eastern Africa you find a diversity of cereals like pearl millet, finger millet, sorghum, barley and wheat. East Africans were hunter gatherers for years. Although this is no longer the case, certain aspects from that lifestyle remain. Collecting nuts and root vegetables to provide energy throughout the day remains a common practice. Hunting is less significant, but meat is still left to cure and dry for later consumption. Raising animals has replaced hunting. Animals like goats, camels, cattle, sheep and donkeys are raised. Livestock is the livelihood for pastoralists and subsistence farmers. Donkeys and cattle are used for tilling the land. Camels are used for transportation. Cattle, sheep, camel and goat are great sources for milk. Milk is used to make butter, cheese, sour milk, and yogurt.

Steamed cooked rice is prepared with spices like cloves, saffron and cinnamon, reflecting historic Persian influence. Soups, lentils and vegetables are usually flavored with curry, thanks to Indian influence. Most meat is marinated with various fruits and spices, then roasted or smoked.

Oranges, lemon and lime are the fruits normally used for marinating.

The Agrarian lifestyle dominates in East Africa. The earliest food crops were sorghum, Bambara groundnuts, cowpeas, yams, and various types of legumes. Trading with South America and Europe over the centuries, impacted agriculture as new crops such as sugarcane, banana, pumpkins, maize, sweet potatoes and cassava were introduced. Maize replaced sorghum. Any farmers' market you go to in urban areas will have maize. Farmers roast fresh maize and sell it to customers.

Food is prepared in creative ways. Maize (corn) may be mixed with legumes and boiled together with a little bit of salt added. A mixture of rice and maize may be enjoyed with sour milk, sprinkled with sugar. Mashed root vegetables like, sweet potatoes, coco yams, or potatoes, may be combined with maize and other legumes.

Ugali is the most significant food in East Africa. It is a moist, sticky dish, made by boiling any sort of flour (maize, sorghum, millet, cassava). Ugali is prepared and served differently and the paste varies in consistency. In Sudan they use coarsely ground maize to make Ugali and enjoy it with sour milk. Sometimes Ugali balls may be wrapped in banana leaves. Ugali is usually served with protein and vegetables. On occasion even peanut butter may be added to Ugali.

In Ethiopia you find the purest indigenous cuisines. The diet is meat based, and they serve it very fresh. Ethiopians prepare food elaborately, taking time to ferment it and spice it with hot peppers. Ethiopians eat *injeral firfir, kichah* (spiced pancake) bread and Ugali (stiff porridge). Ethiopian meals are usually served with a variety of hot sauces.

The hot spiced cardamom tea is popular among East Africans. Cardamom was used to make medicine and perfume in ancient times. Cardamom helped with digestion, relieved urinary complaints, and reduced fever.

Coffee was first discovered in the 9th century in the highlands of Ethiopia. It is believed a goat herder observed his goats acting frisky after eating coffee berries from a bush. In ancient times coffee was used for medicine, food, and beverage. Monks would boil the bean and to help them stay up all night. Coffee was considered an energy laden stimulating fruit.

Traditional Dancing:

In Ethiopia we find the traditional dance Eskesta. This is a shoulder dance performed by Ethiopian Jews. They combine ancient customs, songs, and prayers into a professional dance. Shoulder movement is essential to the art form. The Harlem shake is based on the Eskesta dance.

The Central African Cuisine

Territories:

Burundi
Rwanda
Chad
Congo
Cameroon
Equatorial Guinea
Congo Gabon

History and Food:

Central African food remains for the most part traditional and exotic. Here we also find hundreds of different ethnic groups. The Congo rainforest is the second largest in the world. The ecosystem is as diverse as the people who live there. They have always been hunter gatherers, with a diet based on meat. Centuries ago most of them lived in the forest, and had an unmatched ability to survive there. The men used bows and poison tipped arrows to hunt for meat. Women collected roots, nuts, leaves, mushroom, berries and fruits. They used basic cooking methods, such as roasting, smoking, stewing, and steaming. Families were constantly moving from one campsite to the other. The slave trade in the 16th century introduced cuisines from the outside world, mainly Asia and Europe. However, central African cuisines remain very unique and still prepared in a traditional method. The forests were replaced by farms. The slash and burn agriculture was practiced. The men would cut and burn forests, to create fields for farming, or for livestock. The women did the planting, weeding and harvesting. Beef and chicken are widely enjoyed and other types of game meat.

Meat is usually steamed, boiled, roasted or smoked. Deep-frying is reserved for fish, and this is to preserve it over a period of time without having to refrigerate it. The deep fried fish is normally not breaded or battered. Meat and fish are served with different kinds of sauces. Okra is added to meat dishes to make gumbo. Boiling is the main method of cooking used to prepare sauces. Groundnut peanut sauces are a local favorite adding an interesting taste to meat, and vegetables. Rice, cassava and plantains are the ingredients meals typically consist of.
People eat plenty of salads made up of legumes, meat, fruit and vegetables.

Traditional dance:

The music, dance and culture find its roots in the Ancient "Kongo Kingdom". Here we find the Essombi dance, which depicts warriors preparing for battle, and calling on ancestors and God for strength and courage. Bibunda dance introduces the young girls into womanhood, as they learn to prepare cassava.

Curvy woman cheat sheet
The next pages have a weight loss plan you can follow to lose weight. However, some people are not good at sticking to any plan before they quit or just indulge. Here are some helpful tips to get through the day no matter what phase you are in.

If you had a dream about chocolate or fried foods do not ignore it. Buy or order vitalicious muffin tops and fix your chocolate craving. (vitalicious.com) Enjoy them only on the days you really feel you need chocolate. Eat them with a warm cup of tea with lemon.

Make fried foods at your home. This way you know what you are putting in your body, Use peanut oil, or extra virgin olive oil. Do not reuse any of this oil. Please enjoy fried foods in the afternoon when you are up and about. Don't make it a habit though; you can't eat fried foods constantly. Deep fat frying should be done sparingly. Oven fry your dishes instead.

You cannot have alcohol, sugary drinks, desserts, fried foods and refined carbohydrates in one day! Decide on one indulgence only.

Phase 1

The Hunter- Gatherer/ Subsistence Farmer Phase

In this phase your eating borrows eating habits of both African hunter -gatherers and subsistence farmers. Hunter gatherers eat plenty of berries, roots, fruits, vegetables, lean meats, nuts, and fish. From the subsistence farmers you incorporate the whole grains foods, legumes, dairy, and good oils. This is only for fourteen days. There are five categories to choose food from. Have just one serving size for whatever you choose.

Breakfast: Eat 1 food from category A & 2 foods from category B.

Mid-morning: Enjoy a fruit and veggie smoothie OR Eat 1 food from category D & 1 food from B or a serving of nuts.

Lunch: Eat 1 food from each category.

Evening snack: Enjoy a fruit and veggie smoothie OR eat 2 foods from category D.

Dinner: 4 foods from category E and 1 from category C.

Hunter gatherers have to walk for hours in any given day. Walking is essential to the hunter gatherers lifestyle. You will also need to adopt this behavior. It is easier than you think. Since every step counts I suggest you buy a pedometer. You will need to walk vigorously, at least 45 minutes. This can be broken down into 15 minute increments. In this phase you have to walk for at least 45 minutes every day. Lifting is also essential to the hunter gatherers' lifestyle.

For instance, women lift heavy buckets of water and carry them on their heads for miles. Mirror this by lifting weights for at least fifteen minutes five times a week. Purchase some weight balls and you will see how easy and fun they can be. You will also like the results you get!

Walk schedule
15 minutes brisk morning walk

15 minutes brisk afternoon walk
15 minutes brisk evening walk up a flight of stairs.

Fruit and Veggie Smoothie

Two handfuls of frozen spinach
Two handfuls of frozen Kale
Frozen mixed berries (raspberries, strawberries, blueberries, blackberries,) Optional to select two berries from list.
1 Apple
1 Orange (optional)
½ cup Pineapple or mango(optional)
½ squeezed lime
Cilantro (optional)
½ teaspoon Chia seeds (these seeds help cleanse colon, and get rid of toxins.)
½ tablespoon Flaxseeds (optional)
1 tablespoon sliced almonds (optional)
½ cup water, (add more if needed)

Category A

Breads

1 slice whole wheat bread
½ whole wheat bun or roll
½ whole wheat muffin

½ whole wheat bagel
1 whole wheat tortilla

Rice & Pasta

1 rice cake (any flavor)
½ cup of cooked whole wheat pasta

Waffles & Pancakes

1 whole wheat waffle/organic *
1 whole wheat pancake/ organic
*see basic recipe below

<u>Category B</u>

Dairy

Goat yogurt
Low fat yogurt
Low fat yogurt fruit flavored yogurt *("light" yogurt sweetened with splenda)*
Low-fat 1% milk
Low-fat 2 % milk
Skim milk
Soymilk
Almond milk
Part-skim mozzarella cheese

Parmesan cheese
Low fat cottage cheese
Ricotta cheese
Feta cheese

Protein

Beef jerky (low sodium)
Chicken bacon
Turkey bacon
Pork bacon
Chicken sausage
Turkey sausage
Hard boiled eggs
Scrambled eggs
Poached eggs

Legumes

Canned beans (no sugar added)
Edmame (roasted soybeans)
Soybeans
Pinto beans
Kidney beans
Black beans
Black eyed peas
Chick peas
Split peas
Mung beans
Lima beans

White beans
Butter beans
Lentils
Navy beans
French beans
Green beans
Cowpeas

Fruits

Raspberries
Blueberries
Strawberries
Boysenberries
Cranberries
Blackberries
Grapefruit
Oranges
Apples

Vegetables

Lettuce
Spinach
Green beans
Asparagus
Peppers

Other

Peanut butter *(low fat, omega-3 all natural better option)*

Category C

Meat*

Lean beef
Chicken breasts
Turkey breasts *(low sodium better option)*
Chicken or Turkey sausage
Ground Chicken or Turkey
Lamb
Goat
Liver *(beef or chicken)*

Note: Meat can only be grilled, roasted, steamed, or boiled. Do not add more than a tablespoon of oil to meat dishes.

(*Grass fed meats are best)

Cheese

Cottage cheese
Part-skim mozzarella cheese
Parmesan cheese
Low fat cottage cheese
Part-skim ricotta cheese
Feta cheese

Category D

Note: Fresh fruit & Vegetables only

Grapes
Cantaloupe
Apricots
Pears
Kiwi
Guava
Mango
Passion fruit
Pineapple
Apple
Strawberries
Blackberries
Blueberries
Raspberries
Boysenberries
Cranberries
Honeydew
Peas
Carrots

Category E

Note: Fresh Vegetables only

Cucumber
Mushroom
Broccoli
Cauliflower
Eggplant
Butternut squash
Zucchini
Cabbage
Onions
Celery
Garlic
String beans
Peppers
Tomatoes
Spinach
Leafy greens

Drinks

Water *(drink plenty of water 6-8 glasses a day)*
Herbal tea *(add lemon and lime and a drop of honey for taste)*
Coffee *(sweeten with honey. Don't load your coffee with cream and sugar!)*
Diet organic soda *(with no calories preservatives, sodium or aspartame)*

Nuts 1 serving only *(Roasted or raw no sodium added)*

Almonds
Peanuts
Walnuts
Cashews
Hazelnuts

Fats & Oils *(not more than a serving a day)*

Extra virgin olive oil
Extra virgin coconut oil
Soybean oil
Avocado
Almond butter
Cow's milk butter
Goat's milk butter

Dressings

Homemade organic salad dressings *(see recipe below)*
Annie's organic salad dressings and marinades *(anniesnaturals.com)*

Condiments

Omega 3 mayonnaise

Olive oil mayonnaise
Salsa
Lite salt
Sea salt Light syrup

Dairy Supplements

If you don't enjoy any of the dairy choices, please take calcium supplements every day. Consult your physician as to which calcium supplement to take.

Soups

Use low sodium chicken and beef broth.

Boil and mash the vegetables you like them add the broth to make a soup.
Note: No canned soups.

One week food plan

Monday

Breakfast
1 Slice toasted whole wheat bread
1 Chicken sausage link
Scrambled egg
Glass herbal tea
Calcium supplement

Mid-morning
Fruit and veggie smoothie

Lunch
Grilled pineapple shrimp and whole wheat pasta salad with shredded carrots, sprinkled with soybeans.
Calcium supplement
Herbal tea

Evening snack
¼ Cantaloupe
Blueberries

Dinner
Grilled Sole fish with vegetable stir-fry

Tuesday

Breakfast
1 Whole wheat/organic waffle, strawberries, light syrup
Glass of skim milk

Mid-morning
Fruit and veggie smoothie

Lunch
Whole wheat tortilla chicken wrap, with
spinach and turkey bacon. 1 Mango
Herbal tea
Calcium supplement

Evening Snack
1 Peach
1 Apricot

Dinner
Spinach stuffed tilapia served with grilled
mushrooms.

Wednesday

Breakfast
Whole wheat pancake with light syrup,
strawberries and turkey bacon.

Mid-morning
Yogurt
Blueberries

Lunch
Grilled turkey, (or chicken or beef,) burger
with avocado, cucumber, and lettuce on a ½
whole wheat bun.
1 Orange
Herbal tea

Evening snack
fruit and veggie smoothie

Dinner
Chicken loaf (mix ground chicken with the vegetables and
herbs you enjoy.)
Calcium supplement

Thursday

Morning
1 Slice toasted whole wheat bread
Scrambled egg
Turkey bacon

Mid-morning
Peanuts

1 Glass soymilk

Lunch
½ Bagel pizza with mozzarella and goat
cheese, and sun dried tomatoes, fresh basil.
Serve with pineapple.

Evening Snack
fruit and veggie smoothie
Dinner
Stuffed roasted lamb (lamb roast stuffed with
vegetables)
Calcium supplement

Friday

Breakfast
½ Whole wheat English bagel
1 Turkey sausage
Black beans

Mid-Morning
Cashews
1 Orange

Lunch
Beef chili
Whole wheat tortilla
Tomatoes

Evening Snack
fruit and veggie smoothie

Dinner
Grilled tomatoes and eggplant
Grilled salmon, with mushroom and green
beans.

Saturday

Breakfast
Cheesy scrambled eggs
1 Slice toasted wheat bread

Mid-Morning
Hazelnuts
1 Mango

Lunch

Chicken kabobs
Baked beans
Mushroom and peas stir-fry.
1 Rice cake

Evening Snack
1 Apricot
1 Kiwi

Dinner
Grilled cod served with steamed vegetables.

Sunday

Breakfast
Breakfast burrito, (whole wheat tortilla) with scrambled eggs, chicken sausage, and beans.

Mid-Morning
1 Grapefruit
Walnuts

Lunch
Turkey meatballs
Green salad with carrots and mandarin
oranges
½ Toasted bagel
Calcium supplement

Evening Snack
fruit and veggie smoothie

Dinner
Egg salad
Cup of vegetable soup

Phase 2

<u>The Villager</u>

The villager enjoys organic food from all food
groups. Fresh vegetables are picked from
nearby gardens just before preparation. Fresh

grass fed meat is obtained at the local butcher. In this phase root vegetables are re-introduced into the eating plan. Sweet potatoes, yams, coco yams and red skin potatoes, and rice can be enjoyed once again. In this phase you continue to lose weight. Follow this eating plan until you reach your weight loss goal.

Breakfast: Eat 1 food from category A and 2 foods from category B.

Mid-morning: Fruit and veggie smoothie OR Eat 1 food from category D. Also eat 1 food from B or a serving of nuts.

Lunch: Eat 1 food from each category.

Evening snack: Fruit and veggie smoothie OR 2 foods from category D

Dinner: 4 foods from category E and 1 from category C

Category A

Breads

1 Slice whole wheat bread
½ Whole wheat bun or roll
½ Whole wheat pasta
½ Whole wheat muffin
 ½ Whole wheat bagel
1 whole wheat tortilla

Rice

1 Rice cake *(any flavor)*
½ Rice cooked *(brown rice, basmati rice, and long grain rice)*

Waffles & Pancakes

1 whole wheat waffle/organic *
1 whole wheat pancake/ organic

*see basic recipe below

Root vegetables

Sweet potato
Russet potatoes
Round red potatoes
Yukon potato
New potatoes
Yam
Coco yam

Category B

Dairy
Goat yogurt
Low fat yogurt
Low fat yogurt fruit flavored yogurt *("light"*
yogurt sweetened with splenda)
Low-fat 1% milk
Low-fat 2 % milk
Skim milk
Soymilk
Part-skim mozzarella cheese
Parmesan cheese
Low fat cottage cheese
Ricotta cheese
Feta cheese
Part-skim Ricotta cheese

Protein

Beef jerky *(low sodium)*
Chicken bacon
Turkey bacon
Pork bacon
Chicken sausage
Turkey sausage
Hard boiled eggs

Scrambled eggs
Poached eggs

Legumes

Canned beans (no sugar added)
Edmame (roasted soybeans)
Soybeans
Pinto beans
Kidney beans
Black beans
Black eyed peas
Chick peas
Split peas
Mung beans
Lima beans
White beans
Butter beans
Lentils
Navy beans
French beans
Green beans
Cowpeas
Hummus

Fruits

Raspberries
Blueberries
Strawberries

Boysenberries
Cranberries
Blackberries
Grapefruit
Oranges
Apples

Vegetables

Lettuce
Spinach
Green beans
Asparagus
Peppers

Category C

Meat

Grass fed meats are best
Lean beef
Chicken breasts
Turkey breasts (low sodium better
option)
Chicken or turkey sausage
Ground chicken and turkey
Lamb
Goat
Liver (beef or chicken)

Note: Meat can only be grilled, roasted, steamed, or boiled. Do not add more than a tablespoon of oil to meat dishes.

Fish & Seafood

Tilapia
Hake
Tuna
Crab
Cod
Trout
Fillet of Sole
Haddock
Lobster
Shrimp
Salmon

Cheese

Cottage cheese
Mozzarella cheese
Parmesan cheese
Low fat cottage cheese
Ricotta cheese
Feta cheese

Category D (Fresh fruit & Vegetables only)

Grapes

Cantaloupe
Apricots
Pears
Kiwi
Guava
Mango
Passion fruit
Pineapple
Apple
Strawberries
Blackberries
Blueberries
Raspberries
Boysenberries
Cranberries
Peas & Carrots
Honeydew

Category E

Cucumber
Mushroom
Broccoli
Cauliflower
Eggplant
Butternut squash
Zucchini
Cabbage
Onions
Celery
Garlic

String beans
Peppers
Tomatoes
Spinach
Leafy greens

Drinks

Water (*drink plenty of water 6-8 glasses a day)*
Herbal tea *(add lemon and lime and a drop of honey for taste*)
Coffee (sweeten with honey. Don't load your coffee with cream and sugar!)
Diet soda *(from organic stores with no calories, preservatives, sodium or aspartame)*

Nuts 1 serving only

Note: Roasted or raw no sodium added

Almonds
Peanuts
Walnuts
Cashews
Hazelnuts

Fats & Oils *(not more than a serving a day)*

Extra virgin olive oil

Extra virgin coconut oil
Soybean oil
Avocado
Almond butter
Cow's milk butter
Goat's milk butter

Dressings

Homemade organic salad dressings *(see recipe below)*
Annie's organic salad dressings and marinades *(anniesnaturals.com)*
Condiments

Omega 3 mayonnaise
Olive oil mayonnaise
Salsa
Lite salt
Sea salt Light syrup

Soups
Use low sodium chicken and beef broth
Boil and mash the vegetables you like them add the broth to make a soup.
Note: No canned soups.

Dairy Supplements

If you don't enjoy any of the dairy choices, please take calcium supplements every day.

Consult your physician as to which calcium supplement to take.

Monday

Breakfast
Roasted red skin potatoes
1 Chicken sausage link
Scrambled egg
Glass herbal tea
Calcium supplement

Mid-Morning
Yogurt and Blueberries

Lunch
Rice with stir fry shrimp and broccoli. Served
with baked beans
1 Peach
Calcium supplement
Herbal tea

Evening Snack
Fruit and veggie smoothie

Dinner
Lemon herb roasted chicken breast, with
steamed vegetables.

Tuesday

Breakfast

1 Sweet potato pancake, strawberries, light syrup
Glass of skim milk

Mid-Morning
Almonds
Beef jerky

Lunch
Whole wheat spaghetti & chicken meatballs, sprinkled with parmesan cheese
Green salad
Herbal tea.
Calcium supplement

Evening Snack
Fruit and veggie smoothie

Dinner
Beef and broccoli served with grilled eggplant.
Calcium supplement

Wednesday

Breakfast
Roasted potatoes sprinkled with mozzarella cheese
2 Turkey bacon

Mid-Morning
Yogurt
Blueberries

Lunch
Beef kabobs, (use zucchini, squash, peppers,) served with brown rice, and kidney beans.
1Orange
Herbal tea

Evening Snack
Fruit and veggie smoothie

Dinner
Turkey loaf (mix ground turkey with the vegetables and herbs you enjoy)
calcium supplement

Thursday

Morning
1 Slice toasted whole wheat bread
Scrambled egg
Turkey bacon

Mid-Morning
Peanuts
1 glass soymilk

Lunch
Balsamic lamb chops, served with brown rice,
steamed broccoli,
Fresh spinach & strawberry salad.

Evening Snack
Fruit and veggie smoothie

Dinner
Stuffed roasted chicken breast (roast stuffed
with vegetables like artichoke)
Calcium supplement

Friday

Breakfast
½ Whole wheat English bagel
1 Turkey bacon
1 Poached egg

Mid-Morning
1 Cheese stick
1 Orange

Lunch
Beef stew with vegetables (mushroom, spinach)
Basmati rice
1 Peach.

Evening Snack
Fruit and veggie smoothie

Dinner
Baked stuffed chicken (Stuffed with veggies)

Saturday

Breakfast

1 Slice toasted wheat bread with mozzarella cheese and baked beans

Mid-Morning
Hazelnuts
Blueberries

Lunch
Grilled cod
Sweet potato
Green salad with feta cheese
Mandarin oranges

Evening Snack
Fruit and veggie smoothie

Dinner
Cup of vegetable soup
Grilled shrimp

Sunday

Breakfast
Spinach omelet, whole wheat toast
Herbal tea

Mid-morning
Walnuts
Black grapes

Lunch
Hot turkey sandwich
Salad
1 Fruit *(your choice)*
Calcium supplement

Evening Snack
Fruit and veggie smoothie

Dinner
Chicken vegetable soup

Phase 3

<u>The Modern Villager Phase</u>

Finally you have reached your weight loss goal! You are now a modern villager. You have followed the curvy woman guide and reaped the benefits! At this phase your cravings for junk food have significantly declined. Do not deny yourself completely, no need to kiss chips and cakes goodbye. Occasionally, suitably once a week, go ahead and enjoy a bag of organic chips or brownies. As a modern villager you have access to processed food yet routinely choose organic food instead. Even beer and wine can be enjoyed again.

Breakfast: Eat 1 food from category A and 2 foods from category B.

Mid-morning: Fruit and veggie smoothie OR Eat 1 food from category D and eat 1 food from B or a serving of nuts.

Lunch: Eat 1 food from each category.

Evening snack: Fruit and veggie smoothie OR 2 foods from category D

Dinner: 4 foods from category E and 1 from category C

Note: *Your vegetable intake is not limited. You can add vegetables to any meal. (no root vegetables)*

Category A

Breads and baked goods
1 slice whole wheat bread
½ whole wheat bun or roll
½ whole wheat muffin
½ whole wheat bagel

1 whole wheat tortilla
1 slice homemade cornbread
1 slice cracked wheat bread
1 slice pumpernickel bread
1 whole wheat pita
1 slice rye bread
1 slice raisin bread
1 slice sourdough bread
Low fat homemade blueberry muffin
Low fat homemade bran muffin
Low fat homemade carrot raisin muffin
Low fat homemade corn muffin

Pasta
3/4 Cup cooked whole wheat pasta

Choice of:

Macaroni
Spaghetti
Lasagna
Fettuccine
Angel hair
Rotelle
Linguini
Shells
Spinach pasta
Noodles
Rigati
Fettucine
Lasagna
Wagon wheels
Fusili springs

Grains & Cereal
Amaranth seeds
Oat bran cereal
Granola
Corn bran cereal
Rice bran cereal
Wheat bran cereal
Corn grits

Coucous
Hominy
Millet
Quinoa
Oatmeal
1 rice cake (any flavor)

½ Cup of rice cooked

Choice of:
Brown basmati rice
Long grain brown rice
Wild rice
Jasmine rice
Brown basmati rice
Long grain brown rice
Wild rice
Jasmine rice

Waffles & Pancakes
1 Whole wheat waffle/organic (see basic
recipe below)
1 Whole wheat pancake/ organic

Root vegetables
Sweet potato
Russet potatoes
Round red potatoes
Yukon potato

New potatoes
Yam
Coco yam

Category B

Low fat yogurt
Low fat fruit flavored yogurt (*"light" yogurt sweetened with splenda)*
Goat yogurt
Low-fat 1% milk
Low-fat 2 % milk
Skim milk
Soymilk
Part-skim mozzarella cheese
Parmesan cheese
Low fat cottage cheese
Ricotta cheese
Feta cheese
Part-skim Ricotta cheese
Fromage cheese
Blanc cheese
Swiss cheese

Protein

Beef jerky *(low sodium)*
Chicken bacon
Turkey bacon
Pork bacon
Chicken sausage
Turkey sausage
Hard boiled eggs
Scrambled eggs
Poached eggs

Legumes

Canned beans (no sugar added)
Edmame (roasted soybeans)
Soybeans
Pinto beans
Kidney beans
Black beans
Black eyed peas
Chick peas
Split peas
Mung beans
Lima beans
White beans
Butter beans
Lentils
Navy beans
French beans
Green beans
Cowpeas
Hummus

Fruits

Raspberries
Blueberries
Strawberries
Boysenberries
Cranberries
Blackberries
Grapefruit
Oranges
Apples

Vegetables

Lettuce
Spinach
Green beans
Asparagus
Peppers

Category C

Meat
Note: *Grass fed meats are best*

Lean beef
Chicken breasts
Turkey breasts (low sodium better option)
Chicken or turkey sausage

Ground chicken and turkey
Lamb
Goat
Liver (beef or chicken)
Chicken or turkey thighs, wings, legs (once a week)
Note: *Meat can only be grilled, roasted, steamed, or boiled. Do not add more than a tablespoon of oil to meat dishes.*

Fish & Seafood

Tilapia
Hake
Tuna
Crab
Cod
Trout
Fillet of sole
Haddock
Lobster
Shrimp
Grouper
Halibut
Atlantic herring
Kippered herring
Atlantic mackerel
King mackerel
Spanish mackerel

Mahi-mahi
Monkfish
Ocean perch
Orange roughy
Pollack
Sablefish
Sardines
Swordfish
Salmon

Cheese
Cottage cheese
Mozzarella cheese
Parmesan cheese
Cottage cheese
Ricotta cheese
Feta cheese

Category D (Fresh fruit & Vegetables only)

Grapes
Cantaloupe
Apricots
Pears
Kiwi
Guava
Mango
Passion fruit
Pineapple
Apple

Strawberries
Blackberries
Blueberries
Raspberries
Boysenberries
Cranberries
Peas & Carrots
Honeydew

Category E (Fresh vegetable only)

Cucumber
Mushroom
Broccoli
Cauliflower
Eggplant
Butternut squash
Zucchini
Cabbage
Onions
Celery
Garlic
String beans
Peppers
Tomatoes
Spinach
Leafy greens

Drinks

Water *(drink plenty of water 6-8 glasses a day)*

Herbal tea *(add lemon and lime and a drop of honey for taste)*

Coffee *(sweeten with honey. Don't load your coffee with cream and sugar!)*

Diet organic soda *(with no calories, preservatives, sodium or aspartame)*

Beer and wine once a week

Nuts 1 serving only (Roasted or raw no sodium added)

Almonds
Peanuts
Walnuts
Cashews
Hazelnut
Brazil nuts
Chestnuts
Hickory nuts

Macadamia nuts
Pecans
Pine nuts
Pistachio nuts
Pumpkin seeds
Sesame seeds
Sunflower seed

Fats & oils (not more than a serving a day)

Extra virgin olive oil
Extra virgin coconut oil
Soybean oil

Peanut oil
Sesame oil
Avocado
Almond butter
Argan oil
Cow's milk butter
Goat's milk butter

Dressings

Homemade organic salad dressings *(see recipe below)*
Annie's organic salad dressings and marinades *(anniesnaturals.com)*

Condiments

Omega 3 mayonnaise
Olive oil mayonnaise
Salsa
Lite salt
Sea salt Light syrup

Soups

Use low sodium chicken and beef broth
Boil and mash the vegetables you like them
add the broth to make a soup
Note: No canned soups

Snacks

Baked chips
Popcorn chips
Gourmet air-popped popcorn lightly salted
Rice cakes
Once a week:
Enjoy homemade brownies and cakes
Organic ice-cream
Regular potato chips
Organic chocolate brownie

Monday

Breakfast
Mozzarella, broccoli, and bacon (turkey) omelet
1 Slice whole wheat bread toasted
Cup herbal tea.

Mid-Morning
Almonds
Beef jerky

Lunch
Curry chicken and rice, served with stir-fry vegetables.
Slices of pineapple
Herbal tea
Calcium supplement

Evening Snack
1 Peach
Popcorn

Dinner
Citrus grilled herring served with asparagus, carrots and green beans.

Herbal tea Calcium supplement

Tuesday

Breakfast
Granola with berries and yogurt
1 Cup herbal tea

Mid-Morning
Cashew nuts
1 Orange

Lunch
Shrimp Jambalaya
Strawberry
Spinach tossed salad

Evening Snack
1 Rice cake
1 Kiwi

Dinner
Baked crab and broccoli
Mushroom soup
Herbal tea
Calcium supplement

Wednesday

Morning
1 Pumpkin spice pancake with berries
1 Turkey sausage
Herbal tea

Mid-Morning
Fruit and veggie smoothie

Lunch
Fish curry
Basmati rice
Stir-fry vegetables
Honeydew
Herbal tea

Evening Snack
Popcorn chips

Dinner
Chicken and green bean casserole
Calcium supplement

Thursday

Breakfast
Breakfast burrito (whole wheat tortilla, scrambled eggs, chicken sausage, peppers, onions)
Herbal tea

Mid-Morning
Yogurt with blueberries

Lunch
Beef kabobs (zucchini, red peppers, mushroom)
Sweet potatoes
Green tossed salad
1 Peach

Evening Snack
Fruit and veggie smoothie

Dinner
Blackened grilled salmon
Vegetable soup

Friday

Breakfast
1 Waffle with berries and yogurt

Mid-Morning
Mozzarella cheese stick
1 Mango

Lunch
Oven fried tilapia fish with roast potatoes and carrot
Cucumber salad
1 Plum

Evening Snack
Fruit and veggie smoothie

Dinner
Lemon herb roasted turkey
Steamed vegetables

Saturday

Breakfast
Homemade low fat bran muffin,
strawberries, and
turkey bacon.

Mid-Morning
1 Grapefruit
Pine nuts

Lunch
Grilled chicken and avocado wraps
Coleslaw
1 Peach

Evening Snack
Brownie with ice cream
Herbal tea

Dinner
Cup of vegetable soup.
Shrimp vegetable stir-fry

Best Cooking Styles

Roasting- This is when you cook using dry heat. Most often in the oven in an uncovered pan, or near some hot coals. Food prepared this way usually is very flavorful and low in fat.

Sautéing- This cooking method works best for vegetables such as spinach. Vegetables are cooked and or browned in a skillet or pan containing a small amount of fat over direct heat.

Grilling- Cooking method mainly used for larger chunks of vegetables such as zucchini and eggplant. Also used for meat. Food is cooked over hot coals or other direct heat source.

Blanching- This cooking method is a quick method used for vegetables before freezing them or preparing a dish. Food is placed in boiling water briefly, and then placed in cold water to stop the cooking process. Blanching preserves the color and flavor of vegetables and keeps them crisp.

Steaming- Food is prepared using steam from boiling water. Steaming helps vegetables retain many nutrients.

Boiling- Food is cooked in boiling water or other liquid.

Here are some of my favorite Recipes! Go ahead and try some of them, you will enjoy!

Basic Salad Dressing Recipe

1 tablespoon lemon or lime juice
1/3 cup white or red vinegar
2/3 cup olive oil
½ teaspoon salt
¼ teaspoon black pepper
Pinch of sugar
¼ teaspoon oregano
Grated onion or garlic (optional)

Instructions:
Measure and place all ingredients in a jar or sealed container. Shake well. Allow to refrigerate overnight. Shake well before serving.

African Raisin Rice

Ingredients:
2/3 cup white rice
1level tablespoon curry powder
1 1/3 cup cold water
¼ teaspoon salt
½ cup raisins
Pinch of ground nutmeg
1 tablespoon 100% pure olive oil

Cooking directions:
In a large saucepan cook curry powder in hot oil for 2 minutes. Stir in raisins, rice, water, salt, and nutmeg. Cover with a tight fitting lid. Bring to boil, reduce heat. Cook for 15 minutes and do not lift lid. Remove from heat

after 15 minutes and let stand covered for an additional 10 minutes.

Serve warm. This is delicious with the steak wrapped sausage and a green bean salad.

African Peanut Butter Rice

Ingredients:
2/3 cups brown rice
1 2/3 cup cold water
3 Tablespoons full peanut butter
¼ teaspoon salt

Cooking directions:

In a saucepan bring the rice to boil. Cover saucepan with a tight fitting lid. Reduce heat, and cook for 10 minutes. Remove lid and add the peanut butter. Cover saucepan again and let rice simmer for 10 minutes. Peanut butter will appear bubbly and hot. Stir and mix peanut butter with the rice. Consistency should be semi firm, so you able to roll the rice in your hands. Remove saucepan from heat and let stand with lid on top for 10 more minutes.

Usually served with stews.

African Mutakura

Ingredients:
1 cups dried unsalted peanuts
2 cups corn
2 cup kidney beans
5 cups water

Cooking instructions:
Place all ingredients in a saucepan. Bring to boil. Reduce heat and let simmer until food is soft. Can be enjoyed as a snack.

Chicken Meatloaf

Ingredients:
1 ½ pounds uncooked ground chicken
1 teaspoon sea salt or lite salt
½ large onion finely grated
2 tablespoons olive oil
½ cup of whole wheat cracker crumbs
(optional)
Fresh thyme chopped
1 clove garlic minced
Fresh mushroom finely chopped

Directions:
Preheat oven to 375 degrees.
Mix all ingredients except the olive oil. Mix until evenly combined. Place into loaf pan and shape. Pour olive oil over the loaf. Bake for 40-45 minutes until the top is a golden brown. Cool before serving. Slice and serve.

Low Fat Egg rolls (25 egg rolls)

Ingredients:
2 pounds lean ground organic chicken, turkey or organic beef sausage. (If you substitute for ground chicken, turkey or beef add the spices you like)
1 packet coleslaw mix (can substitute with grated carrots and shredded cabbage.)
4 fresh basil leaves,
3 fresh sage leaves,
Finely grated onion (optional)
Finely grated red bell peppers.
1 packet egg roll wrappers
100% extra virgin olive oil
Sweet and sour chili sauce (can use fish sauce instead)
½ cup hot water
Romaine lettuce

Cooking instructions:
Place meat in a saucepan and add ½ cup hot water. Allow meat to cook, and brown it. Add onions and stir in for about a minute. Add coleslaw, basil, sage, and red peppers. Stir in for about two minutes, so vegetables are lightly cooked. Remove from heat and allow cooling. Following the directions included in

the egg roll wrapper package, make individual rolls with the mixture.

Wrap egg rolls in lettuce and dip in chili or fish sauce. Enjoy!

Beef Jerky, Edamame (soybean) and Raisin Snack.

Ingredients:
1 packet Beef jerky (preferably low sodium.)
½ cup Roasted soybeans
1 tablespoon raisins

Cut beef jerky strips into bite size pieces.
Place beef jerky into sandwich bag.
Add roasted soybeans and tablespoon raisins.
Enjoy as a snack anytime

Eastern African Cardamom Tea

What you need:
6 cups Cold water
4 teaspoons (Breakfast English tea, Earl Grey, etc)
Ground cardamom
Honey
Milk (optional)

What to do:
Heat the water in a saucepan or teakettle to a near boil.
Transfer the water to a teapot and add the tea leaves.
Pour tea into cups, add a pinch of cardamom, sugar, or honey to taste. Stir. Serve with meal.

Low Carb Pizza

Ingredients:
3 whole wheat low carb tortillas
1 cup chopped pineapple
3 organic chicken sausages any flavor
¾ cup Marinara sauce
Fresh basil
¾ cup Mozzarella cheese
Dried Oregano
Tomatoes, onions, garlic (optional)

Directions:
Preheat oven to 350 degrees
Place whole wheat tortillas on baking trays.
Cover each tortilla in marinara sauce.
Sprinkle mozzarella cheese.
Remove sausage from casing. Make little balls and place on tortillas. Layer chopped pineapple on top of sausage. Sprinkle oregano. Chop fresh basil and sprinkle on top. Bake for 20- 25 minutes. Enjoy!

Sadza

Ingredients:
2 -4 cups mealie meal or white corn meal
1 cup Water or beef broth

Directions:
In a saucepan with a lid bring to boil 4 cups of water.
In a bowl make a thick paste with 3 cups of the mealie meal and 3 cups of water. Set aside 1 cup for use later.
Slowly add the paste to the boiling water stirring all the time, to prevent lumps. Stir for a few minutes on medium high heat. Slowly add the rest of the mealie meal to the pot until sadza is thick and smooth.
Reduce heat to low, let cook for a few minutes.

Zimbabwean Chicken Stew - Serves 4-6

What you need:

2 pounds fresh boneless chicken breasts cut into bite size cubes
3 large carrots chopped,
handful of green beans sliced
3 ripe red tomatoes cubed
Olive oil to fry
1 bunch spring onions, sliced
1 medium chopped onion
1 ginger, skinned and finely sliced
1 tsp black pepper
1/2 tsp chili powder
1 red chili paste
1 tsp salt
1/2 tsp dried parsley

What to Do:
To make tomato sauce, heat olive oil in a large saucepan over medium heat. When oil is hot stir-fry the ginger for 30 seconds. Add the onions and continue to stir-fry. Add the chili paste

and enough chili powder to redden the onions.
Still stirring continuously, add

the black pepper and then the salt. Sprinkle
the dried parsley into the pot. Turn the heat to
high and add the chopped tomatoes a little at
the time (keep the mixture boiling all the
while).
When you have added all the tomatoes turn
the heat down to medium and simmer for ten
minutes. Add carrots and green beans; turn the
heat down to low and cook for 15 minutes.
In a frying pan heat olive oil. Brown chicken
on both sides. When evenly browned add to
the sauce already made in the saucepan.
Simmer for 25 minutes, stirring occasionally.
Serve with sadza, rice or couscous.

Oxtail Soup Recipe

Ingredients:
Serves: 4-6
3 lbs. oxtail (Fat trimmed off) 1/4 cup oil
cups water
2 tomatoes, chopped
2 onions, chopped
1 clove garlic, chopped
2 teaspoons dried thyme
1 cup chopped carrots
1 packet fresh mushrooms
2 teaspoons dried sage
2 red grated peppers
1 heaped teaspoon Sea salt
Coarse ground pepper

Directions:
Brown oxtail in oil. Stir in some of the chopped onion, and grated red pepper. Season with sea salt and black pepper. Add 5 cups of water and boil. When there is no more water, pour out any excess fat. Stir in tomatoes, sage, thyme, and the rest of the onions and peppers. Add 5 more cups of water and let oxtail simmer for about 2 hours or however long it takes to make them tender. When oxtail is

tender add carrots and mushroom and let simmer until vegetables are cooked.

Best served with rice and peas.

Ugandan Mango and Pumpkin Soup

Ingredients:

1 Small chopped pumpkin or large can of pumpkin
6 ripe mangos
4 to 5 cups of water
1 cup low fat plain yogurt
¼ cube of butter
1 teaspoons ginger powder
5 small low sodium vegetable bouillon cubes
I tsp paprika
1 tsp rosemary leaves
1 chopped onion
Minced parsley
2 big teaspoons minced garlic

Directions:
In a saucepan heat the butter and add onions, ginger, and garlic and sauté on low heat for 5 minutes.
Add ginger powder, bouillon cubes, paprika, and rosemary leaves and the water and cook on low heat for 20 minutes. Remove skin from mangoes, cut off the fruit and put in blender. Blend then set aside.

Blend pumpkin mixture for 7 seconds. Add the mangoes to the pumpkin mixture, add yogurt, and cook for ten more minutes. Garnish and serve hot or cold with salad and bread.

Serves 6-8

African Fish Curry

Ingredients:
3 pounds tilapia or cod
Olive oil spray
1 cup coconut milk
1 large chopped onion
2 teaspoons of curry powder
Tamarind paste or powder to taste
3 tomatoes chopped
2 sweet green peppers chopped
6 garlic cloves minced

Directions:
Lightly brush fish with olive oil and grill it to brown both sides, and not to cook it. Place fish in a saucepan, and cover in coconut and tamarind. Set aside. Stir together the onion, tomatoes, garlic, spices, and green pepper. Add to the fish and coconut milk. Simmer slowly on low heat until fish is fully cooked, and sauce is thickened. Serve on a bed of rice.

Moroccan Carrot, Orange & Radish Salad

6 servings

Ingredients:
1 lb Carrots, peeled & shredded
2 tablespoons Lemon juice
1 Large Onion, chopped
2 tablespoons Orange juice
3/4 cup radishes, thinly sliced
1/2 cup cilantro, chopped
3 tablespoon Olive oil
Salt and pepper
Pita wedges
Dash of cinnamon

In a salad bowl combine carrots, radishes, oranges, and
cilantro. Whisk together the olive oil, juices, salt and pepper and pour over the salad. Cover & chill. Serve
garnished with pita wedges.

Algerian Chicken Coriander

Ingredients:
5 boneless chicken breasts,
4 tablespoons olive oil
4 large cloves of garlic crushed
1 teaspoon turmeric
Sprig of fresh coriander leaves, (finely chopped) or 2 teaspoons ground coriander,
1 lemon sliced
Handful of purple olives, pitted

Directions:
In heavy skillet heat oil, add chicken and brown it. Add garlic cloves, coriander, and spices. Cook for about ten minutes. Stir in enough water to cover the food and simmer over low heat until the chicken is tender. Add olives and lemon and simmer for 8-10 more minutes. Serve over couscous

Before 210 pounds

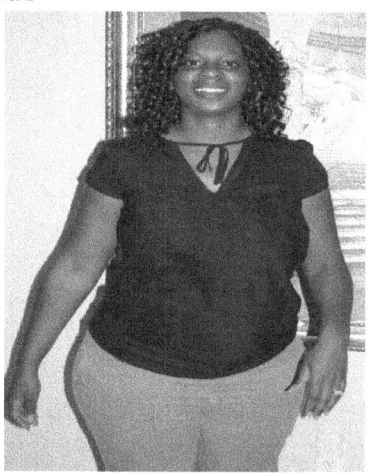

My little sister Danai Salerno, lost weight, but look below she kept her curves!

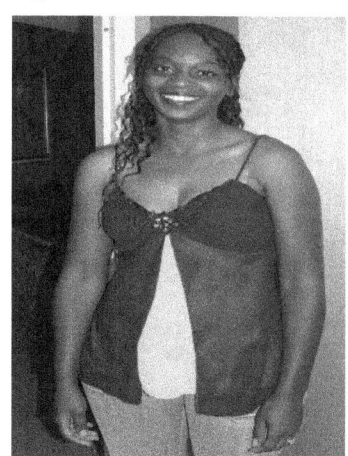

After 140 pounds

Curvy Women this is your time! Success to your weight loss goals and much joy to you.